DIABETES
A Whole Foods Plant-based Approach

EDWARD ESKO
ALEX JACK
BETTINA ZUMDICK

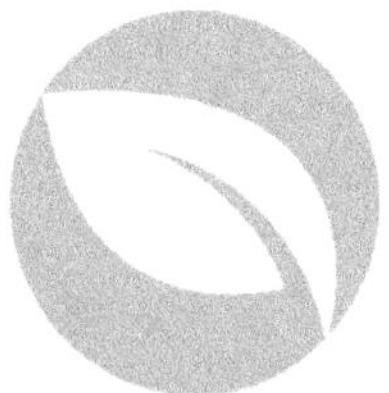

Berkshire Holistic Associates
PLANT BASED NUTRITION & LIFESTYLE

"Our research, funded by the National Institutes of Health, has shown that a healthful plant-based diet has a dramatic effect on diabetes. It helps people improve their blood sugars, lose weight, cut their cholesterol and blood pressure, and reduce their medication use. And sometimes the disease disappears altogether. Instead of trying to manage the disease with medication, the first approach should be to tackle its cause—which is on our plates."*

—Neal D. Barnard, M.D., FACC
Adjunct Associate Professor of Medicine, George Washington University School of Medicine; President, Physicians Committee, Washington, DC

"In 2009 the macrobiotic center in Massachusetts hosted a weeklong workshop for type 2 diabetes. The participants were introduced through lectures to the effects of diet, obesity, stress and the lack of exercise on the body resulting in the development of "metabolic syndrome." This is defined as "excess body fat around the waist, increased blood pressure, high blood sugar, and abnormal cholesterol or triglyceride levels all occurring together which increases the risk of heart disease, diabetes and stroke."

"Weights were taken initially as well as blood pressures and blood sugars. These measurements were repeated mid-week and at the end of the week. During the course of the week, dietary changes were initiated which was a macrobiotic diet emphasizing plant based, no dairy, no simple sugars, no meat except fish once or two times a week, whole grains, and a variety of vegetables. In addition, cooking classes were offered, and daily exercise scheduled. Discussion groups were held and individual consultations offered.

"Over the course of the week, we saw a weight loss of an average of three pounds, blood sugar levels dropped, as did blood pressure measurements to the extent that medication had to be reduced. Participants reported an increase in energy and expressed their increased sense of well-being. One woman in particular, who was having a great deal of difficulty walking—

having to stop every few feet to catch her breath—was by the end of the week walking without difficulty. She was absolutely amazed as were the rest of the participants.

"It was a most successful and encouraging experience for all, including me, the attending physician."
—Martha Clayton Cottrell, M.D.

"We are entering an exciting new period in healthcare where holistic practices are being integrated with western medicine. Current trends are moving away from the limiting symptoms-based approach of diagnosis and treatment to an encompassing patient-centered approach. Plagued by unanswered questions and unsuccessful treatments that can lead to other issues, such as unwanted side effects and dependency, western physicians and patients are looking for ways to address all aspects of illness including the root cause.

"In addition, each day more physicians and patients are acknowledging the impact food and lifestyle has on the development of illness. New scientific studies repeatedly reveal the benefits of eating a primarily plant-based diet, and the field of epigenetics has shown how food, meditation and lifestyle affect gene expression. Mind, body and spirit all play a role in wellness, and these factors impact sickness and health to a much larger degree than once believed. Management and treatment have begun to focus on a comprehensive approach using multiple healing modalities.

"Macrobiotics provides a foundation for diagnosing and treating illness, as well as explanations for why people have conditions and how they can overcome them. It identifies the constitution, or genetic predisposition of a person, as well as the current condition. Tools such as visual diagnosis are used that lead to a deeper understanding and connection with the patient. Macrobiotics also emphasizes that healers use intuition to guide their patients to health, and it teaches the importance of healing from within as well as the steps to do so."
—Sommer White, M.D.

"This document on diabetes is clear and simply elegant. The Dao (Tao) doctrines have been practiced in Asia for over 7,000 years unifying the concept of yin and yang. This document explains the basic concept of yin and yang and how foods, body organs, and metabolism fit into the balancing of the two major forces to keep our bodies healthy.

"All of us will develop different degrees of diabetes as we age as the pancreas beta cells will age and our bodies will have a decreasing ability to utilize glucose efficiently. If you incorporate some of the regimen of using whole grains and vegetables recommended, your chances of developing clinical diabetes will decrease.

"Try it you will feel the difference as the best proof of truth. The scientific references are well studied and confirm its effects. Show them to your doctors. I encourage donors to support this proposed study as it is not only about diabetes but also about chronic diseases such as cancer."
—George Yu, M.D.

DIABETES
A Whole Foods Plant-based Approach

Contents

New Berkshire Study to Offer Whole Foods to Diabetes Patients

Berkshire residents with Type 2 Diabetes will have the opportunity to participate in a Whole Foods, Plant-Based Intervention medical wellness study this year. The disease, which affects almost 12% of Americans, is largely a dietary and lifestyle-mediated disorder linked to the standard American diet high in processed animal foods, sugar and other refined sweeteners, and other ultra-processed foods and beverages.

Conducted by Berkshire Holistic Associates, a division of the nonprofit Planetary Health, Inc., and approved by the Berkshire Medical Center, the study will assess whether a balanced macrobiotic diet, a popular form of plant-based nutrition, provided to individuals with type 2 diabetes, improves blood glucose control and reduces use of insulin and other hypoglycemic medication. Mark Pettus, M.D. of Berkshire Health Systems in Pittsfield will serve as principal investigator and the three of us will serve as co-investigators. Donna Clifford, R.N. will be available as on-call nurse.

The out-patient study would include pre- and post-intervention assessment for 10 to 15 local, primarily Berkshire County residents with type 2 diabetes referred by their primary care physicians in the community. The study would extend over a period of 6 weeks and include an educational component consisting of weekly cooking classes and lectures at Eastover Resort & Eco-Village in Lenox. Local and national food companies will be asked to donate whole grains, beans, vegetables, seasonings, condiments, and other specialty items for use in the study and would be provided free to participants to improve compliance with the study's dietary guidelines.

Eligibility for the study would be subjects 18 years or older who have a medically confirmed diagnosis of type 2 diabetes and who are undergoing pharmacological treatment with insulin and/or glucose-lowering medications. They will complete a macrobiotic dietary therapy course, consisting of 12 hours of practical cooking classes (selection of food items, amounts, combinations, proportions, eating frequency, handling, cooking methods, and food preservation), and 12 hours of theory (principles underlying the diet and its nutritional and therapeutic potential) for implementation on their own at the end of the study.

Principal investigator Dr. Mark Pettus, an internist and nephrologist practicing for more than 25 years, commented:

"This is one of the first direct dietary intervention studies for diabetes in the United States," explained Alex Jack, president of Planetary Health, Inc. and author of *The Cancer Prevention Diet, Diet for a Strong Heart*, and other popular books. "If successful, it could serve as a template for other communities throughout the country."

Edward Esko, author of *Diabetes: The Macrobiotic Approach* and director of the International Macrobiotic Institute, added: "With the mounting evidence linking diet with the cause, prevention, management, and potential recovery from diabetes, the time has come for clinical trials of the macrobiotic approach. Macrobiotics could very well offer a solution to this 21st century epidemic."

Bettina Zumdick, author of *Authentic Foods* and founder of the Culinary Medicine School in Lee, further noted: "In my history of working with clients I have witnessed dramatic improvements and recoveries from diabetes type II, which resulted in an overall improvement of health and quality of life of the individuals. It is wonderful and exciting to be part of conducting this study which can potentially mean a tremendous difference in someone's life and as a downstream effect in many people's lives."

In a recent article "Our Food Is Killing Too Many of Us," Dariush Mozaffarian, dean of the Tufts Friedman School of Nutrition Science and Policy, and Dan Glickman, former U.S. Secretary of Agriculture, declared that poor diet is the leading cause of mortality in the U.S. "More than 100 million adults—almost half the entire adult population—have pre-diabetes or diabetes. Cardiovascular disease afflicts about 122 million people and causes roughly 840,000 deaths each year, or about 2,300 deaths each day. Three in four adults are obese. More Americans are sick, in other words, than are healthy." They called for "Food Is Medicine" solutions, including patient prescription programs for healthy produce and nutrition education in elementary, middle, and high schools to address the health crisis.

Speaking English is not a requirement for the Berkshire study. Volunteer interpreters and translators will be sought to assist non-English speakers as much as possible. No stipends will be provided to participants. However, in kind food donations by natural foods communities could be worth $500 to $1000 per participant in the course of the study. A modest $10/week travel allowance will also be budgeted per participant to defray gas and mileage to classes in Lenox.

The study was approved this autumn by the Institutional Review Board of Berkshire Medical Center in Pittsfield, the principal hospital in the region. We three co-investigators are longtime macrobiotic teachers and dietary counselors and for the study completed a certified course in medical ethics. Berkshire Holistic plans to raise $25,000 for the study through individual and corporate donations, as well as grants and online crowdsourcing. Tax-deductible donations may be sent to Planetary Health, Inc., Box 487, Becket MA 01223.

Alex Jack, Edward Esko, and Bettina Zumdick
The Berkshires
November 21, 2019

Understanding Diabetes
Edward Esko

According to estimates, diabetes is positioned to become the leading public health epidemic of the 21st century. Worldwide, the incidence of diabetes has increased dramatically. Diabetes is expected to affect 350 million people by 2030, doubling from the 2000 level of 170 million. The greatest increase is expected to occur in the developing countries of Asia, Africa, and the Persian Gulf.

In the United States, the number of people with diabetes jumped from 5.6 million in 1980 to 20.9 million in 2010. Close to 27% of persons over age 65 now have diabetes. One in three Americans are predicted to develop diabetes by mid-century. The cost of treating diabetes in the U.S. will soon approach $200 billion per year. Diabetes threatens to overwhelm health care systems in this country and around the world. Diabetes is a major factor in the ongoing financial crisis caused by skyrocketing health care costs.

Modern medicine remains powerless in the face of this planet-wide surge. In a special 200th anniversary article in the *New England Journal of Medicine* (*NEJM* 2012; 367-1332/October 4, 2012) entitled "The Past 200 Years in Diabetes," Dr. Kenneth Polonsky states: "…The pathway to cure has remained elusive. In fact, if one views diabetes from a public health and overall societal standpoint, little progress has been made toward conquering the disease during the past 200 years, and we are arguably worse off now than we were in 1812."

Could it be that after billions in research and decades of effort, we are worse off now than we were two centuries ago? Perhaps it is time to take stock and reassess. Perhaps a fresh approach is called for. Let us now examine diabetes from the macrobiotic perspective, beginning with the role of the pancreas.

The Role of the Pancreas

The pancreas is a flat shaped organ located on the left side of the body below the stomach. In its structure, function, and energy it is complementary to the liver, the large organ located opposite it on the right side. The pancreas, being lower in position and more flat than the liver, is classified as yang. The liver, being larger and more expanded, is comparatively yin. (Yang is the term used to describe smaller or more compact forms; yin is the term used to describe larger, more expanded forms.)

The pancreas is animated primarily by celestial force flowing down toward earth. This more yang force is stronger on the left side of the body. The descending colon is evidence of its influence. The liver, on the other hand, receives stronger upward energy. This more yin force originates with the rotation of the earth and is stronger on the right side of the body. Hence the ascending colon is located on the right. The primary forces of yin and yang create the organs and animate their respective functions.

This classification is essential and relevant to our understanding of the cause of diabetes as well as to the prevention and recovery from this disease.

Looking at the way in which these organs interact to regulate the level of glucose (sugar) in the blood will help illustrate this further. The metabolic sugar cycle is divided into stages:

1. Eating food
2. Digesting, or breaking carbohydrate down into glucose (simple sugar)
3. Glucose entering the blood
4. Pancreas releasing insulin
5. Glucose exiting blood and entering body cells.

The processes of eating, digestion, and the absorption of glucose by the bloodstream represent the yin or expansive phase of the cycle. Chewing and digestion are processes of breakdown and decomposition, in this case, breaking down more complex carbohydrates into simple sugar known as glucose. The release of insulin by the pancreas and the entrance of glucose into the cells are the yang or contractive phases in the cycle. The net result of the yin phase is a rise in blood glucose (sugar), while the result of the yang phase is a decrease in blood glucose. High blood sugar is yin, while low blood sugar is yang.

Insulin & Glucagon are synthesized in pancreatic islet cells

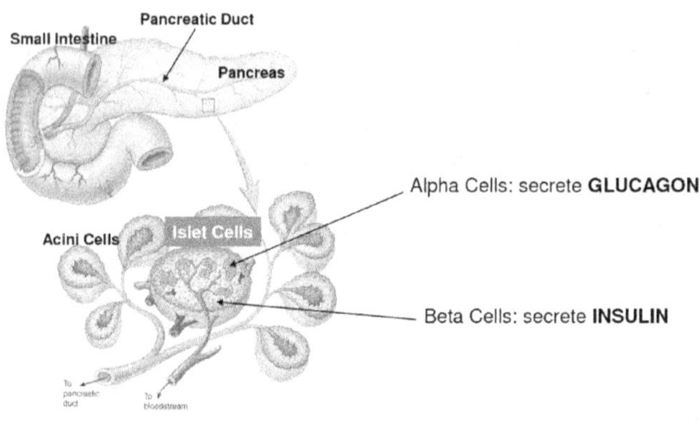

The pancreas performs a dual function. The acini cells secrete digestive enzymes, similar to saliva. On the whole, pancreatic digestive juice is alkaline and yang. It especially aids in the digestion of fats, which are yin.

Scattered throughout the pancreas are about a million cell clusters known as the "islets of Langerhans." The islets are a compact collection of endocrine cells that secrete the hormones that regulate the conversion of sugar into energy and hence the level of sugar in the blood.

The two primary endocrine cells are known as alpha cells and beta cells. The smaller and denser beta cells secrete the yang hormone insulin, which lowers blood sugar. Alpha cells, which are larger and more expanded, secrete the yin hormone glucagon, which has the effect of raising the level of sugar in the blood. As we saw above, on the whole the pancreas is a yang organ. The pancreas contains far more beta cells than alpha cells. The ratio of beta cells to alpha cells is approximately 85% to 15%, or about seven parts beta to one part alpha.

Insulin and Glucagon

Insulin and glucagon offer a perfect example of complementary balance. When blood sugar becomes elevated, the beta cells secrete insulin. Insulin causes glucose to enter the body's cells, thus lowering the blood sugar level. It also signals the liver to bind glucose molecules for storage in the form of glycogen. The net result is a decrease in blood glucose.

Conversely, when the glucose level becomes low, the alpha cells secrete glucagon. This yin hormone signals the liver to break stored glycogen (yang) down into free glucose (yin), thus raising blood sugar levels.

The mechanism by which insulin facilitates the entry of glucose into the body's cells can also be understood in terms of yin and yang. Cells consist of an outer cell membrane (yin) and an inner cell nucleus (yang.) Free glucose circulating in the blood is yin, while insulin, as we saw, is yang. Glucose is naturally repelled by the yin cell membrane; it needs a yang agent to facilitate transfer through the membrane and into the interior of the cell. This is accomplished by insulin.

Insulin readily bonds with receptors on the cell membrane and passes through the membrane into the interior. The presence of insulin below the surface membrane changes the quality of the membrane. It now becomes yang and attracts and admits glucose.

What is Diabetes?

Diabetes occurs when the pancreas either does not produce enough insulin or when the body's cells resist or reject the insulin that is produced. The result is high blood sugar, or hyperglycemia, which produces a number of symptoms and side effects, both immediate and long term. In his article Dr. Polonsky describes the disease as follows:

"Over the past two centuries, we have learned that diabetes is a complex, heterogeneous disorder. Type 1 diabetes occurs predominantly in young people and is due to selective autoimmune destruction of the pancreatic beta cell, leading to insulin deficiency. Type 2 diabetes is much more common, and the vast majority of people with this disorder are overweight. The increase in body weight in the general population, a result of high-fat, high-calorie diets and a sedentary lifestyle, is the most important factor associated with the increased prevalence of type 2 diabetes. Older adults are most likely to have type 2 diabetes, although the age at onset has been falling in recent years. Type 2 diabetes is now common among teenagers and young adults.

"We now know that insulin resistance is essential in the pathogenesis of type 2 diabetes, and that the disease results from both insulin resistance and impaired beta cell function."

Both insulin resistance and impaired beta cell function are yin conditions, as are obesity and overweight. A primary cause of these conditions is the intake of strongly yin simple sugars, such as refined sugar, as well as refined carbohydrates like white rice and white flour.

The continual intake of extremes exhausts and depletes the beta cells. The result is either not enough insulin or insulin that is too weak to facilitate the transfer of glucose across the cell membrane. If insulin lacks strong yang power, it will not be

able to bond with the cell membrane and enter the interior of the cell. Without insulin as a facilitator, glucose does not enter the cell but remains circulating in the blood, hence the high level of blood glucose characteristic of diabetes. This mechanism explains the onset of type 2 diabetes.

The mechanism of type 1 diabetes is a little different, albeit also extremely yin. T. Colin Campbell, Ph.D. in *The China Study*, best describes the process:

This devastating, incurable disease strikes children, creating a painful and difficult experience for young families. What most people don't know, though, is that there is strong evidence that this disease is linked to diet and, more specifically to dairy products. The ability of cow's milk protein to initiate type 1 diabetes is well documented.

In some infants, cow milk proteins are not fully digested and small amino acid chains or protein fragments are absorbed by the small intestine. In the bloodstream the immune system identifies these fragments as antigens, or foreign proteins, and codes antibodies to destroy them. Some of these protein fragments are identical in form to insulin-producing beta cells. Antibodies produced by the immune system thus destroy both the cow proteins and the beta cells, taking away the child's ability to produce insulin. The result is type 1 diabetes, an incurable lifetime condition.

Once again, we can understand this process in terms of yin and yang. Milk, a product of the yang animal body, is a powerfully yin secretion designed for growth. This is especially true for the milk of large mammals such as cows. The intake of this strongly yin substance (often together with refined sugar) is largely responsible for the onset of type 1 diabetes.

Good Carbs vs. Bad Carbs

Carbohydrates come in two types: "simple" or "complex." Simple carbohydrates contain just one sugar molecule (monosaccharide) or two sugar molecules (disaccharide). Simple sugars demonstrate strong expansive force. These yin molecules enter the bloodstream very quickly. They cause a rapid spike in blood sugar. In contrast, complex carbohydrates consist of a chain of sugar molecules linked together. Their strong bonding force is yang. The body has to work harder to break down the links in the chain; hence they enter the bloodstream more slowly than simple sugars. The level of sugar in the blood remains more constant and steady. This distinction is crucial in understanding the effect of diet on diabetes.

Simple Carbohydrates

monosaccharide (glucose)

disaccharide (sucrose)

Complex Carbohydrates

polysaccharide

Examples of simple carbohydrates include table sugar, honey, fruit, fruit juice, jam, and chocolate. They are often labeled "bad" because they are high in calories compared to their nutritional content and because of their effect on blood sugar. Complex carbohydrates are lower in net calories and are sometimes touted as "healthy carbs." They include foods like whole grains, beans, whole grain bread and pasta, vegetables, especially sweet-tasting ones, and sea vegetables.

A1c

Yin and yang can help us understand how the A1c test works. The A1c test is used to measure levels of blood sugar and the appearance of diabetes. The test is based on a measurement of the amount of sugar, or glucose, that attaches to red blood cells. At their core, red blood cells contain hemoglobin; a protein that contains iron and that carries oxygen from the lungs to all the cells of the body. Because of their hemoglobin, and the iron it contains, red blood cells are strongly yang. Thus red cells readily attract and bind with oxygen, which is yin. Iron is a dense, solid, and heavy metal; oxygen is a light yin gas. Red cells also link up with sugars such as glucose, which as we have seen, are also yin. Glucose (yin) enters the red blood cells and binds (or glycates) with molecules of hemoglobin (yang), an example of the law of opposites attracting. The higher the level of glucose in the blood, the more hemoglobin gets glycated. Measuring the percentage of A1c in the blood makes it possible to get an overview of average blood glucose levels over the previous two to three months.

The normal range for the hemoglobin A1c test for persons without diabetes is between 4% and 5.6%. Increased risk for diabetes is reflected in hemoglobin A1c levels between 5.7% and 6.4%. A level of 6.5% or higher indicates diabetes. These levels indicate the red cells have lost their normal yang quality and are becoming yin—over expanded and weak.

Studies have repeatedly shown that uncontrolled diabetes results in complications from the disease, such as eye, kidney, skin, and other potentially serious problems. Doctors advise people with diabetes to achieve a hemoglobin A1c that is less than 7%. Healthy A1c levels can be achieved by eliminating white sugar, white bread, white rice, and white potato and by adopting a balanced macrobiotic diet.

Brown vs. White Rice

Organic brown rice contains beneficial fiber, minerals, vitamins, and phytochemicals like beta-carotene.

Milling and polishing brown rice removes most of its vitamins and minerals. It also strips away most of the fiber in brown rice. The fiber in brown rice and other whole grains slows the absorption of glucose and helps prevent diabetes. That is because the carbohydrate in whole grain fibers is yang and cohesive. The body has to work harder to break the links that bind the carbohydrate chains together.

Although the starch in white rice, white flour, and a baked potato is in the form of complex carbohydrate, the body converts this starch into blood sugar almost as quickly as it pro cesses pure glucose. These foods cause a rapid rise in blood sugar and are classified as having a high glycemic index. The glycemic index classifies foods on how quickly and how high they raise the level of sugar in the blood in comparison to pure glucose.

As we have seen, a food like brown rice is digested more slowly. It doesn't cause a rapid spike in blood sugar and is classified as having a low glycemic index. When brown rice is milled and refined by removing its bran and germ, its glycemic index rises. The same is true of whole wheat and other grains. Finely ground grain (yin or expansive) is more rapidly digested than coarsely ground grain (more contractive or yang), and has a higher glycemic index.

The type of starch is also a factor in determining a food's glycemic index. More yin starches, like those in potatoes, are rapidly digested and absorbed. Potatoes have a high glycemic index.

More yang starches, like those in brown rice, are processed more slowly and have a low glycemic index. Because of these factors, brown rice is being touted as a possible solution to the diabetes epidemic, especially in China and other rapidly developing countries. A January 2012 article from the Harvard School of Public Health entitled, "Can Brown Rice Slow the Spread of Type 2 Diabetes?" states:

"The worldwide spike in type 2 diabetes in recent decades has paralleled a shift in diets away from staple foods rich in whole grains to highly refined carbohydrates, such as white rice and refined flours. Now a group of researchers at Harvard School of Public Health (HSPH) aims to stem the tide by changing the color of the world's rice bowl from white to more-nutritious brown."

The announcement of a collaborative initiative to prevent the global diabetes epidemic by improving the quality of carbohydrate consumed follows an earlier study published on June 14, 2010 on the website of the journal *Archives of Internal Medicine*. In the study, HSPH researchers found that eating five or more servings of white rice per week was associated with an increased risk of type 2 diabetes, while a diet that includes two or more servings of brown rice was associated with a lower risk.

The investigators estimated that the risk of type 2 diabetes could be lowered by 16% by replacing 50 grams of white rice (1/3rd of a typical daily serving) with the same amount of brown rice. Interestingly, replacing the same amount of white rice with whole wheat or barley was associated with a 36% lower risk.

"From a public health point of view, whole grains, rather than refined carbohydrates, such as white rice should be recommended as the primary source of carbohydrates fro the U.S. population," said senior researcher Frank Hu. "These findings could have even greater implications for Asian and other populations in which rice is a staple food."

The Potential of Plant-based Diets

Macrobiotic educators have for decades advocated an approach similar to the approach advocated by the Harvard School of Public Health. The macrobiotic diet may offer the most effective approach to the prevention of diabetes. Macrobiotics advocates avoiding milk and dairy products associated with type 1 diabetes. Breast-feeding is the preferred method of

nourishing infants and children. Refined sugar and artificial sweeteners like high fructose corn syrup are not recommended. Macrobiotics recommends avoiding or reducing foods such as potatoes, white flour, white rice, and others with a high glycemic index. Instead, foods rich in complex carbohydrates and fiber like whole grains, beans, fresh vegetables, and sea vegetables are the foundation of the macrobiotic diet. These foods are associated with a lower risk of type 2 diabetes. The quality of salt used as seasoning is also important. Mineral rich sea salt is preferred over refined table salt. Some evidence has come in that one brand of sea salt, known as Si Salt, harvested in the pristine ocean off Baja California, aids in lowering blood sugar levels.

Moreover, the macrobiotic diet may prove an effective tool in the management of diabetes. In type 2 diabetes, successful management and recovery have been noted in persons adopting a macrobiotic way of eating. Persons with type 2 diabetes have experienced a marked reduction in the need for medication; some after only one or two weeks after beginning the diet.

Some patients have eliminated the need for medication entirely while noting marked improvements in overall health. At the very least, macrobiotics is acknowledged as an effective tool in weight loss and weight management. Patients with type 1 diabetes have noted reductions in the need for insulin and a lessening of complications after adopting a plant-based macrobiotic way of eating. Macrobiotics can help these patients better manage their condition.

With the mounting evidence linking diet with the cause, prevention, management, and potential recovery from diabetes, the time has come for clinical trials of the macrobiotic approach. Macrobiotics could very well offer a sustainable solution to this 21st century epidemic.

Whole Foods, Plant-based Intervention Study for Type 2 Diabetes

Alex Jack

Introduction

Over 30 million Americans—1 in 8 Americans—are diagnosed with diabetes, the fastest growing chronic disease in the country, and nearly 300 million people around the globe have the condition. According to the World Health Organization, the number of cases will double by 2030. Diabetes contributes to increased death and disability from heart disease, stroke, kidney disease, blindness, and amputations. Meanwhile, the cost of treatment is rising, resulting in added burden to individuals, families, and society. According to the American Diabetes Association, health care costs associated with diabetes rose from $174 billion in 2007 to $245 billion in 2012, an increase of 41% in five years. Medical expenditures for people with diabetes are 2.3 times higher than people without the disease and are the main driver for the increased overall financial burden on the country. 20% of all health care expenses in the country go to the care of people diagnosed with diabetes. It is widely recognized that lack of physical activity, stress, and poor nutrition, especially the intake of highly processed foods, sugar, soft drinks, and fried foods are factors contributing to this trend.

Dietary intervention can help prevent, control, and in some cases relieve diabetes, among both adults and children. The macrobiotic way of eating, a whole-foods dietary approach introduced by educators including Michio and Aveline Kushi based on whole cereal grains, beans, vegetables from land and sea, and other fresh, largely unprocessed or traditionally processed foods, is especially beneficial. Scientific and medical studies have documented its benefits, as described below. In recognition of the contribution of macrobiotics to American health and well being, the Smithsonian Institution has established a permanent Michio Kushi Collection on Macrobiotics at the National Museum of American History in Washington, D.C.

Berkshire Holistic, an educational charity based in Massachusetts and part of the nonprofit Planetary Health, Inc., has designed a dietary intervention study that is aimed at improving the health and well being of adults with Type 2 diabetes. In the future, the dietary principles and practices of this pilot program could be expanded to include juvenile or Type 1 diabetes. If successful, the project could be offered to families, schools, hospitals, and schools, significantly improving the health and well being of the American people and serving as a model for other regions.

The Plant-based Macrobiotic Approach

During the last half century, macrobiotics has been in the forefront of the worldwide health and diet revolution, serving as the catalyst for many of the dietary and lifestyle changes now circling the globe. Macrobiotics has introduced modern societies organically grown whole foods and naturally processed foods, including brown rice, whole wheat, and other whole grains; miso, tofu, tempeh, and other traditional soy products; a cornucopia of fresh garden vegetables; wakame, kombu, and other sea vegetables; and a variety of high-quality seasonings, condiments, and sugar- and dairy-free desserts and snacks. Macrobiotics has also popularized holistic health and alternative and complementary methods that are now embraced by millions of people and by the medical profession.

"Macrobiotics" comes from *makro bios*, the Greek words for "Long Life" and "Great Life." Hippocrates, the Father of Medicine, coined the term and in the modern era Michio Kuahi and other educators in America, Europe, and Japan have developed it.[1] By creating our minds and bodies from whole natural foods in a spirit of thankfulness, we can contribute to personal health, social well being, and planetary health and peace.

The benefits of a macrobiotic diet are widely recognized today, as the scientific and medical studies noted below show. From a tiny seed in the 1960s, macrobiotic principles have blossomed, nourishing society at many levels. In the early 1970s, research on the macrobiotic community at Harvard University and the Framingham Health Study identified dietary cholesterol and saturated fat as major risk factors in the development of heart disease. The scientists also found that individuals observing a macrobiotic way of eating (on average for 2 years) had the healthiest blood values of any group ob served in modern society. [2]

The landmark dietary and nutritional changes over the last generation have been influenced and shaped by macrobiotics, from the historic report *Dietary Goals for the United States* by a Select U.S. Senate Committee in the late 1970s to the U.S. Government's Food Guide Pyramid in the 1980s, from the creation of the Office of Alternative Medicine within the National Institutes of Health in the 1990s to the shift toward a plant-centered diet and the primacy of whole grains in the 2000s.

The changes that took place constituted a nutritional axis shift. The Four Food Groups—based on meat and dairy food—were replaced with a more balanced way of eating centered on grains, vegetables, fruits, and other plant foods. As the new century began, the U.S. Dietary Guidelines accompanying the Food Guide Pyramid called upon Americans to "use plant foods as the foundation of your meals":

There are many ways to create a healthy eating pattern, but they all start with the three food groups at the base of the Pyramid: grains, fruits, and vegetables. Eating a variety of grains (especially whole grain foods), fruits, and vegetables is the basis of healthy eating. Enjoy meals that have rice, pasta, tortillas, or whole grain bread as the center of the plate . . . .

Eating plenty of whole grains, such as whole grain bread or oatmeal, as part of the healthful eating patterns described by these guidelines, may help protect you against many chronic diseases. [3]

The benefits of a macrobiotic way of eating have been recognized by the major scientific and medical societies and published in leading journals, including the *New England Journal of Medicine, Journal of the American Medical Association, American Journal of Clinical Nutrition,* and many other publications.[4]

Studies on Diabetes

• A study by the Ministry of Public Health in Thailand in 2006 found that a macrobiotic way of eating offers an effective, alternate approach to the care of diabetes patients and that it may help patients on insulin maintain their blood sugar levels without an insulin injection. In a dietary intervention study at the Wanakaset Research Facility of Kasetart University in Trad Province, researchers introduced a special macrobiotic diet to 44 type 2 diabetes patients, including four on insulin. For a period of between two and fourteen weeks, the subjects were required to refrain from using drugs and chemicals and to observe a balanced macrobiotic diet.

At the end of the program, the researchers found a statistically significant reduction in blood sugar levels, weight, blood pressure, and heartbeat ratios.

"Subjects were in significantly better health, more vibrant, more peaceful, and more energetic," the study reported. The four patients on insulin were able to maintain their blood sugar levels within the range of 110-171 mg without any insulin injections and all subjects were free of any adverse effects. 85.7 percent of subjects reported better health compared to a year earlier and 81 percent reported better emotional status for the same period. "The results of the present study can be a guideline in the modification of health care policies that can lead to the development of effective, and alternative care of diabetes mellitus patients," the researchers concluded.[5]

• In a 6-month macrobiotic dietary intervention study carried out in 16 adults with Type 2 diabetes at the Diabetic Care Center in Colon in 2009, Cuban physicians reported that anthropometric variables significantly improved, including lean body mass and glucide and lipid metabolism. "All participants were able to eliminate insulin treatment, and 25 percent continued treatment with glibenclamide only," the researchers reported. Mean total cholesterol, LDL cholesterol and triglyceride values dropped 16.4, 22.7, and 37.0 percent respectively, while mean HDL cholesterol rose 97.8 percent. Mean glycemia and HbA1 values also decreased 63.4 and 54.5 percent respectively. "According to lipid levels and ratios, cardiovascular risk was also considerably reduced." The investigators noted. "Hemoglobin, total protein, albumin, and creatinin levels indicated that nutritional safety was maintained. There were no adverse events."[6]

• In a review of the macrobiotic approach to diabetes and other chronic diseases, Robert H. Lerman, M.D., Ph.D., noted, "eating a diet high in fiber potentially reduces the risk for cardiovascular disease and diabetes mellitus." He cited a recent case series in 13 patients with type 2 diabetes provided with nutrition education and provided with meals at the Kushi Institute in 2010.

Under the supervision of Martha Cottrell, M.D., most experienced reduction in or elimination of diabetes medication, weight loss, reduced blood pressure, and improvement in energy after starting the new way of eating in the course of the program.[7]

• Physicians Committee for Responsible Medicine (PCRM) conducted an experiment in which 99 individuals with type 2 diabetes were assigned to a low-fat vegan diet for 22 weeks. Dr. Neal Barnard, the president of PCRM and a supporter of the macrobiotic approach, reported in 2006 that overall the subjects were able to control their blood sugar three

times more effectively than the control group that adhered to the American Diabetes Association Diet. Both groups experienced weight loss, lower plasma lipid levels, reduced urinary albumin excretion, and lower hemoglobin A1c (measuring

---

blood sugar levels over time), but those in the vegan group also experienced greater reductions in A1c, weight, body mass index, waist circumference, total cholesterol, and LDL cholesterol.[8]

• The role of brown rice and other whole grains in the these studies was underlined several years ago in a study that grew out of the Framingham Study, the oldest continuous study of diet and heart disease in the United States and one that has long evaluated and promoted the macrobiotic approach to cardiovascular health. In a cross-sectional study of 2941 overweight subjects in the Framingham Offspring Study cohort, USDA researchers at Tufts University in Boston reported in 2002 that whole-grain intake was inversely associated with body mass index, total cholesterol, LDL cholesterol, and fasting insulin, while consumption of refined grains did not benefit the overweight participants. "Increased intakes of whole grains may reduce disease risk by means of favorable effects on metabolic risk factors," the scientists concluded.[9]

• In Africa, researchers with the Black Women's Health Study reported in 2006 that women who consume millet, barley, and other whole grains high in magnesium might reduce their risk of type 2 diabetes by up to one-third.[10]

• Two years earlier, New Zealand scientists reported in 2004 that people who consume about 3 servings per day of whole grain foods are 20 to 30 percent less likely to develop type 2 diabetes. "There is strong evidence to suggest that eating a variety of whole grain foods and legumes is beneficial in the prevention and management of diabetes," the researchers observed.[11]

• Seaweed, an important part of the daily macrobiotic way of eating, has been shown to expand in the stomach and slow the digestion of food, resulting in lower blood glucose spikes after a meal. In a case-control study of diabetic patients in Korea published in 2008, subjects in the seaweed supplementation group ingested 2.5 times as much fiber as the control group. Fasting blood glucose levels and 2-hour postprandial blood glucose measurements decreased significantly in those ingesting seaweed. Triglyceride levels also fell, HDL cholesterol rose, and other metabolic risk factors also improved. "Ingestion of seaweed influences glycemic control, lowers blood lips, and increases antioxidant enzyme activities," the researchers concluded.[12]

• In a randomized case control study of 76 obese patients with impaired glucose tolerance and type 2 diabetes, Japanese researchers added kanten, a traditional plant-based gelatin made of seaweed and a staple in the macrobiotic way of eating, to the experimental group and reported that mean reduction of body weight, BMI values, and total cholesterol were lower in the agar group than in the conventional controls. "The agar diet resulted in marked weight loss due to the maintenance of reduced calorie intake and to an improvement in metabolic parameters," the scientists concluded in their 2005 report.[13]

• In short- and medium-term trials conducted on patients with type 2 diabetes, Italian researchers concluded that the Ma-Pi2 diet, a macrobiotic diet developed by Mario Pianesi, significantly improved indicators of metabolic control, including fasting blood glucose, glycosylated hemoglobin, the serum lipid profile, body mass index, body weight and blood pressure. The diet may also alter the gut microbiota composition, which could additionally affect glycemic control. "As a result, the Ma-Pi 2 diet could be considered a valid additional short- to medium-term treatment for T2DM."[14]

• In a follow up study, Italian researchers collected the stools before and after intervention from a subset of forty par ticipants with Type 2 diabetes, in order to measure the gut microbiota rRNA sequencing and metagenomics. As a comparison, the gut microbiota of 13 normal-weight healthy controls were evaluated. The scientists found that both diets were effective in modulating gut imbalances in diabetic subjects, resulting in an increase of the ecosystem diversity and supporting the recovery of a balanced community of health-promoting microorganisms. The macrobiotic diet, but not the control diet, was also effective in counteracting the increase of possible pro-inflammatory groups, such as Streptococcus, in the gut ecosystem, showing the potential to reverse pro-inflammatory conditions, and possibly explaining the greater efficacy in improving the metabolic control.[15]

The Planetary Health Study

The purpose of the PHI/BHS Study is to assess whether in individuals with Type 2 diabetes, a balanced macrobiotic diet improves blood glucose control and reduces use of insulin and other hypoglycemic medication. The principal measure is hemoglobin A1c. Cardiovascular risk factors and dietary acceptability are also assessed.

Participants would be enrolled from diabetics who would commute or stay at a residential facility to receive daily meals and periodic classes. The study duration is 6 weeks with several medical checks and follow up, including a voluntary weekly support group for patients/participants.

The study will be held under the auspices of Berkshire Medical Center, the primary healthcare hospital in the region and patients would be referred by primary care physicians. The sample size is based on the studies described above and the expected difference between the baseline measurements and the intervention diet outcomes.

Primary Outcome Measures
• Hemoglobin A1c [Time frame: 6 weeks]

Secondary Outcome Measures
• Body weight [Time frame: 6 weeks]
• Plasma lipid concentrations [Time frame: 6 weeks]
• Blood pressure [Time frame: 6 weeks]
• Urinary albumin [Time frame: 6 weeks]
• Dietary Acceptability [Time frame: 6 weeks]

• Serum vitamin D [Time frame: 6 weeks]
• Serum high specific C-reactive protein
• BMI changes [Time frame: 6 weeks]

Follow Up
• Subjects would be tested for the above variables after completion of the initial study after 6 months and again after 12 months

Enrollment   10 to 15 subjects

Eligibility
Eligible Ages   18 years and older
Gender   All
Healthy Volunteers   No

Inclusion Criteria
• Confirmed diagnosis of Type 2 diabetes
• Voluntary participation with informed consent
• Pharmacological treatment with insulin and hypo- or normo-glycemic tablets, or both
• Residence at or near the dietary intervention center in Becket, MA, including participation in daily meals prepared by trained cooks at Eastover Resort & Eco-Village in Lenox, Massachusetts
• Completion of a macrobiotic diet therapy course, consisting of 12 hours of practical cooking classes (selection of food items, amounts, combinations, proportions, eating frequency, handling, cooking methods, and food preservation) and 12 hours of theory (principles underlying the diet and its nutritional and therapeutic potential) for implementation when they return to home cooking at the end of the three-month study. Participants would be asked to en-

courage their spouse, partner, or other family member to take the dietary therapy course and assist with subsequent cooking. Participants would be encouraged to participate in some exercise and get adequate exposure to the natural environment

Exclusion Criteria
• Hemoglobin A1c values <6.5% or >10.5%
• Use of insulin for >5 years
• Tobacco use within the preceding 6 months
• Consumption of more than 2 alcoholic beverages per day
• Current drug abuse
• Pregnancy
• Unstable medical status
• Current use of a low-fat, vegetarian, vegan, or macrobiotic diet

The study will be conducted according to the guidelines described in the Declaration of Helsinki and the Institutional Review Boards of the participating medical center will approve all procedures involving human subjects/patients.

Location
Eastover Resort & Eco-Village, Lenox, Massachusetts

Sponsors
Berkshire Holistic Associates
Planetary Health, Inc.

Staff
Principal Investigator: Mark Pettus, M.D.

Education and Counseling Directors: Edward Esko, founder of the International Macrobiotic Institute, Alex Jack, President of Planetary Health, Inc.; Bettina Zumdick, founder and director of the Culinary Medicine School

Medical Consultants: Sommer White, M.D., Martha Cottrell, M.D., George Yu, M.D., Lynn Chittick, R.N., and other physicians or health care practitioners to be decided.

Meal Supervision: Macrobiotic Summer Conference and International Macrobiotic Institute Food Service Coordinators and Instructors, including Bettina Zumdick, Naomi Ichikawa Esko, and others.

A Plant-based Macrobiotic Approach

The macrobiotic diet is a plant-based, seasonally- and locally-oriented approach to nutrition. Foods grown organically are preferred over those raised chemically. GMOs are avoided whenever possible.

The proposed diet consists of about 40-50 percent by weight of whole cereal grains (brown rice, millet, barley, etc., 30-40 percent vegetables (onions, carrots, pumpkin, squash, broccoli, cauliflower, kale, red and white radish, parsley, etc.), beans and bean products (chickpeas, lentils, adzuki beans, tofu, tempeh, etc.), sea vegetables (wakame, kombu, nori, etc.), fermented products (miso, shoyu, umeboshi, etc.), seasonings and condiments (sea salt, sesame seed salt, etc.), natural grain-based sweeteners (rice syrup, barley malt, amasake, etc.), and natural spring or well water, bancha twig tea (tannin-free green tea), and other non-stimulant, nonaromatic beverages. A small volume of fish or seafood would be available for those who desired animal products. As much as possible, food would be fresh, organic, and locally grown or processed.

Study participants will receive full food service daily (breakfast, lunch, dinner and snacks) in the macrobiotic dining hall. Expert macrobiotic cooks will prepare food. Patients may have more than one serving as long as proportions of grains, vegetables, and legumes are maintained.

Budget

Total to be determined, including project administration, food costs, medical supervision and testing, nutrition education, and tuition, room, and board for participants.

Project Staff and Consultants

Alex Jack is President of Planetary Health, Inc. and senior macrobiotic teacher and counselor. He is the co-author with Michio Kushi of *The Macrobiotic Path to Total Health* (Ballantine, 2003), *Diet for a Strong Heart* (St. Martin's Press, 1985) and *The Cancer Prevention Diet* (St. Martin's Press, 2009), and with Aveline Kushi of *The Complete Guide to Macrobiotic Cooking* (Time-Warner, 1985).

Edward Esko is the Founder and President of the International Macrobiotic Institute in Massachusetts. He is the founder of Berkshire Holistic Associates in Lenox, Mass. He is the co-author with Michio Kushi of *Holistic Health Through Macrobiotics* (Japan Publications, 1993), *Macrobiotic Cooking for Everyone* (Japan Publications, 1980), and *Basics and Benefits of Macrobiotics* (One Peaceful World Press, 1995).

Bettina Zumdick, founder of the Culinary Medicine School in Lee, Mass., has been involved in macrobiotics for over twenty-five years. A native of the Baltic Sea area in Germany, she studied food science at the University of Muenster. Bettina has taught macrobiotics and other mind-body-spirit related topics such as meditation, Tao Yin Yoga and chanting throughout Europe and the United States. She is the author of *Authentic Foods.*

Sommer White, M.D. worked as an ER physician in Los Angeles. After graduating from the Kushi Institute Leadership Training Program, she moved to Nashville, Tenn., where she has an integrative/macrobiotic medical practice.

Martha Cottrell, M.D. has given seminars on diet and diabetes at conferences and gatherings around the world. The former medical director of the Fashion Institute of Technology in New York City, she is the co-author with Michio Kushi of *AIDS, Macrobiotics, and Natural Immunity* (Japan Publications, 1990) She lives in Asheville N.C.

George Yu, M.D. is a professor of surgery at George Washington University Medical School in Washington, D.C. He has participated in many medical studies on macrobiotics, diet and health, and holistic approaches to cancer, cardiovascular disease, and diabetes.

Conclusion

It is hoped that the proposed study will show that the macrobiotic way of eating can be successfully implemented among the general American public and significantly improve the health and well-being of persons with Type 2 diabetes, as well as reduce obesity and the risk of cardiovascular disease, improve productivity, and substantially reduce mounting health care costs. It could lead to further studies, including trials with children and adolescents suffering from this affliction, as well as serve as a template for similar studies across the country or around the world.

Case Studies

Ken Becker

About three or four years ago, I began to look for alternatives to the conventional medical way of treating my diabetic condition, which I had had for about six years. I found it hard to accept the conclusion that because of my condition I would have to live my whole life as a "sick" man. A little over one year ago, my search was rewarded: I discovered macrobiotics, a system that not only offered me hope, but actually started to heal me in front of my own eyes!

I undertook macrobiotics as a skeptic, and only my own practical experiences have convinced me of its effectiveness. The thing that impressed me most about macrobiotics was not only that it *worked*, but also that it provided me with an explanation of *why* I had diabetes—something conventional medicine had been unable to do—and of how my body would react and change as it began to heal itself. I was amazed at how accurate these predictions were. In eight months, just as predicted, my body's requirement of insulin was reduced by one half, from about 40-42 units per day to about 18-20 units per day.

Even more impressive was the dramatic improvement in my overall health. As any medical doctor and every diabetic knows, diabetes has an effect on the person's general health: circulation is impeded, susceptibility to colds and infections increases, eyesight deteriorates, muscle tone is harder to maintain, and so forth.

Before becoming diabetic, I was a fairly healthy child. Afterwards I watched as my health deteriorated in these and many other ways. All of these complications have disappeared since I've become macrobiotic, and my general good health is returning.

I have not had a cold since becoming macrobiotic (my previous average was 4-5 per year), a 7-year case of red, sore throat has disappeared (my doctor had told me "that's just the

way you are"), a 7-year long case of running nose has ban-
ished, my eyesight has improved, I have no more headaches,
my gums no longer bleed when I brush my teeth, my previ-
ously poor complexion is a thing of the past, I no longer get
muscle cramps and nervous twitches—the list could go on and
on. Some of these improvements could be attributed to the improvement in my diabetic condition, but I believe they are all
directly related to my change in eating.

Source: *Cancer and Diet*, East West Foundation, Brookline, Mass, 1980.

Peter Howes

I went for a consultation with Mr. William Tara at the Community Health Foundation in London in September 1977 to
talk about my diabetic condition, and was given a specific
macrobiotic diet to follow. The difficulties of preparing the
macrobiotic meals were overcome by gradually incorporating
the new foods into our normal family diet. After four weeks I
was completely on the new diet, and found the transition from
the established habits of a lifetime much easier than I had an-
ticipated. At first I experienced some stomach pains, but these
have not recurred.

I occasionally craved for the foods I used to enjoy. (I
would wake up in the night with my mouth watering at the
thought of dried fruits, oranges and bananas!) But these crav-
ings soon passed, and not the only remaining desire is for an
occasional glass of beer. I do not give into this, though, for
fear of once again becoming a drinker, with the accompanying
problem of excess liquid.

The most amazing development over the last nine months
has been a new state of quietness and calm. My sleeping habits
have also become more regular: I am usually in bed by 11, and
awake completely refreshed at 5:30. Before my change in diet

I was useless until 10 in the morning and my first cup of coffee—on which I was dependent throughout the day!

Now about nine months after beginning macrobiotics, my insulin requirement has been reduced by about one half, and I find that my condition is easier to control, since the tendency to swing from high blood sugar to low blood sugar has been stabilized by my new diet. My weight has also reduced, and I feel very fit and full of energy.

Source: *Cancer and Diet*, East West Foundation, Brookline, Mass, 1980.

Macrobiotic Diabetes Project

In 2009 Kushi Institute brought together a medical doctor, Martha Cottrell, M.D., a videographer, researcher, and 13 people diagnosed with and on medication for type 2 diabetes. This week was designed to explore the positive effects of a macrobiotic diet and lifestyle on type 2 diabetes. Results of the project were remarkable, with many participants being able to dramatically reduce their medication, and some even eliminating medication by the end of the week! Additional benefits included experiencing greater vitality, mobility, and feelings of well-being.

I attended a macrobiotic seminar and lost 22 pounds and my blood sugar level is almost normal. My doctor supports my decision to stop my medication saying that I'm doing as well or even better off the medicine. Five weeks after attending your program I'm continuing to do great. Thank you Kushi Institute and macrobiotics. — David Woodin

Source: KushiInstitute.org.

Larry Bogoslaw

I had always liked sweets, and I had a problem with bed-wetting since I was four, but I never had any real problems with my health until October 1972 when I was eight years old. I remember the night of my cousin's bar mitzvah. I hadn't eaten all day, and I was so hungry by the end of the evening that I binged on as much cake as I could eat. The next morning I threw up and began to feel really fatigued. My mother took me to a paediatrician and the diagnosis was hype 1 diabetes; I was put on one shot of insulin per day.

I lacked the willpower to stay on the structured diet plan I was given. By the time I was eleven another doctor put me on two shots of insulin a day in an effort to better control my blood sugar, since I wasn't eating as carefully as I was supposed to. From the start, I was always a very undisciplined eater and drinker, and very poor at following any doctor's instructions; in fact, developing the ability to be orderly and disciplined in my approach to taking care of myself has been one of the biggest changes I have experienced now in my year of practicing macrobiotics. I recall always being angry in the first few years. I had cut sugar out of my diet, but I was still eating plenty of meat.

In 1980 my father discovered macrobiotics in Philadelphia through the East West Foundation. Although my father began eating a macrobiotic diet, I didn't begin until I came to Boston in June 1983, where I had my first macrobiotic consultation and was given a completely different way to eat right away. At this time I was taking 65 units of insulin a day. Marc Cauwenberghe, the consultant I saw, told me I could possibly be taking as little as 5 or 10 units of insulin by the end of the summer, and I was sure he was crazy! After about ten days of eating a macrobiotic diet I was able to decrease my insulin dosage, dropping by 10% increments, from 65 units to 46 units. By June 20th it was down to 35 or 40 units, and some time in July it went down to 30. Early in August, an experienced macrobiotic cook moved into the apartment where my father and I were staying, and after a short period of eating her cooking, my insulin suddenly took another leap downwards.

In addition to the decrease in my insulin intake, I soon noticed a number of other changes. My acne diminished to a few small, dull bumps on my cheeks, and my complexion was brighter; my shoulders were suddenly straighter; and my energy calm and consistent from 8 a.m. to midnight. As the weeks became months these changes were accentuated, and

---

more deep-seated transformations became apparent as well. Most importantly, it became clear that one old, deeply ingrained assumption of mine was no longer true. This was the assumption that I would not live past the age of thirty-five. With the constant feeling of my vitality ebbing away, every year and every month, this was a constant background in my awareness and approach to life. Now my daily insulin dosage is down to about 15 units, my vitality is ever increasing, and I am enjoying every minute of it, since I know that all my dreams, all my potential will be realized. If I can change this much in a year, anybody else can change too!

Source: KushiInstitute.org.

Macrobiotics
Plant-based Dietary and Way of Life Suggestions
For persons living in a temperate climate

Daily Dietary Recommendations

WHOLE CEREAL GRAINS. Between 40 and 50% by weight of every meal is recommended to include cooked, organically grown, whole cereal grains prepared in a variety of ways. Whole cereal grains include brown rice, barley, millet, whole wheat, rye, oats, corn, and buckwheat. Please note that a portion of this amount may consist of noodles or pasta, unyeasted whole grain breads, and other partially processed whole cereal grains.

SOUPS. 1-2 cups or bowls (about 5-10%) of your daily food intake may include soup made with vegetables, sea vegetables (wakame or kombu) grains, or beans. Seasonings are usually miso or shoyu (organic soy sauce.) The flavor should not be too salty.

VEGETABLES. About 25-30% of daily intake may include local and organically grown vegetables. Preferably, the majority is cooked in various styles (e.g. sautéed with a small amount of vegetable oil, steamed, boiled, and sometimes as raw salad or naturally fermented or pickled vegetables.

Vegetables for daily use include green cabbage, kale, broccoli, cauliflower, collards, pumpkin, watercress, Chinese cabbage, bok choy, dandelion, mustard greens, daikon greens, scallion, onion, daikon, turnip, various   fall   and   summer squashes, burdock, carrot, varieties.

Avoid or limit the intake of potato (including sweet potato and yam), tomato, eggplant, pepper, spinach, asparagus, beet, zucchini, and avocado. Mayonnaise and other oily, fatty, or artificial dressings are best avoided.

BEANS AND SEA VEGETABLES. ¼ to ½ cup (about 5-10%) of the daily diet may include cooked beans and sea vegetables. Beans for regular use include azuki, chickpea, lentil, and black soybean, as well as kidney, navy, black bean, white beans, pinto, non-GMO soybean, and others. Bean products such as tofu, tempeh, and natto can also be used. Sea vegetables such as wakame, nori, kombu, hiziki, arame, dulse, agar, and others may be prepared in a variety of ways. They can be cooked with beans or vegetables, used in soups, or served separately as side dishes or salads, moderately flavored with brown rice vinegar, sea salt, shoyu, ume plum, and other natural seasonings.

OCCASIONAL FOODS. Animal quality food is optional. If needed or desired, 1-3 times a week, approximately 10% of the daily consumption of food can include fresh wild caught flaky white meat fish. Non-farm raised salmon and sea scallops can be included several times per month if your condition permits.

Fruit or fruit desserts, including fresh, dried, and cooked fruits, may also be served three or four times per week on average. Local and organically grown fruits are preferred. If you live in a temperate climate, avoid tropical and semi-tropical fruit and eat, instead, temperate climate fruits such as apples, pears, plums, peaches, nectarines, apricots, berries, and melons. Local organic fruit juice may also be consumed if your condition permits.

Lightly roasted nuts and seeds such as pumpkin, sesame, and sunflower may be enjoyed as snacks, together with peanuts, walnuts, almonds, and pecans.

Rice syrup, barley malt, amasake, and mirin may be used as sweeteners, together with occasional maple syrup. Brown rice vinegar, lemon, or umeboshi vinegar may be used for a sour taste.

BEVERAGES. Recommended daily beverages include bancha (kukicha) twig tea, stem tea, roasted brown rice and barley tea, and occasional dandelion and corn silk tea. Any traditional tea that does not have an aromatic fragrance or a stimulating effect can be used. You may also drink a comfortable amount of water (preferably spring or well water of good quality) but not iced.

FOODS TO REDUCE OR AVOID. Meat, animal fat, eggs, poultry, dairy products (including butter, yogurt, ice cream, milk, and cheese), fatty fish and seafood, refined sugars, chocolate, molasses, honey, other simple sugars like stevia, agave, evaporated cane juice, etc., and foods treated with them.

Tropical or semi-tropical fruits and fruit juices, including banana and pineapple, soda, artificial drinks and beverages, coffee, colored tea, and all aromatic stimulating teas such as mint or peppermint.

All artificially colored, preserved, sprayed, or chemically treated foods, including foods with GMO ingredients. All refined and polished grains, flours, and their derivatives. Mass-produced industrialized food including canned, frozen, and irradiated foods.

Hot spices, any aromatic stimulating food or food accessory, artificial vinegar, and strong alcoholic beverages, especially those produced from sugar or mixed with sugared beverages.

ADDITIONAL SUGGESTIONS

Cooking oil should be vegetable quality only, with natural cold pressed olive and sesame as preferred varieties.

Salt should be naturally processed sea salt. Traditional, non-chemical shoyu or tamari soy sauce and miso may be used as seasonings.

Recommended condiments include:

—Gomashio (sesame salt made from approx. 20 parts roasted sesame seeds to one part sea salt)

—Sea vegetable powder or flakes, including green nori, dulse, kelp, wakame and others, as well as combinations or blends

—Sesame seed wakame powder

—Umeboshi plum

—Tekka

—Roasted seeds such as sunflower or pumpkin

Pickled vegetables made without sugar or strong spice, including non-pasteurized organic sauerkraut, pickled Chinese cabbage, and others may be eaten on a daily basis.

You may have meals regularly, 2-3 times per day, as much as you want, provided the proportion is correct and the chewing is thorough. Avoid eating for approximately 3 hours before sleeping.

THE IMPORTANCE OF COOKING. Proper cooking is very important for health. Everyone should learn to cook either by attending classes or under the guidance of an experienced macrobiotic cook. The recipes included in macrobiotic cookbooks may also be used in planning meals.

SPECIAL ADVICE

The guidelines present above are general suggestions. These suggestions may require modification depending on your individual condition. Of course, any serious condition should be closely monitored by the appropriate medical, nutritional, and health professional.

Together with beginning to change your diet, we invite you to attend regular seminars, cooking classes, and study programs and to meet with a qualified macrobiotic counselor or educator.

Way of Life Suggestions

- Live each day happily without being preoccupied with your health; try to keep mentally and physically active.
- View everything and everyone you meet with gratitude, particularly offering thanks before and after each meal.
- Chew your food very well, at least 50 times per mouthful, or until it becomes liquid.
- It is best to retire before midnight and get up early every morning.
- It is best to avoid wearing synthetic or woolen clothing directly on the skin. As much as possible, wear cotton, especially for undergarments. Avoid excessive metallic accessories on the fingers, wrists, or neck. Keep such ornaments simple and graceful.
- Take a ½ hour walk each day. When safe and appropriate, walk barefoot on grass, beach, or soil. Keep your home in good order, from the kitchen, bathroom, bedroom, and living quarters, to every corner of the house.
- Initiate and maintain an active correspondence, extending your best wishes to parents, children, brothers and sisters, teachers, and friends.
- Avoid taking long hot showers or baths unless you have been consuming too much salt or animal food.
- To increase circulation, scrub your entire body with a hot, damp towel very morning or every night. If that is not possible, at least scrub your hands, feet, fingers and toes.
- Avoid chemically perfumed cosmetics. For care of the teeth, brush with natural, fluoride-free preparations.
- If your condition permits, exercise regularly as part of daily life, including activities like walking, scrubbing floors, cleaning windows, washing clothes and working in the garden. You may also participate in exercise programs such as yoga, martial arts, dance, or sports.

- Avoid using electric cooking devices (stoves, ovens, ranges) or microwave ovens. Convert to gas cooking at the earliest opportunity.
- It is best to minimize the use of color television, computer monitors, cellphones, tablets, smartphones, and other mobile devices.
- Include large green plants in your house to freshen and enrich the oxygen content of the air in your home. Open windows frequently to permit air to circulate freely.
- Sing a happy song every day.

Special Dishes and Remedies
Specific for Diabetes

The recipes in this section have special benefits for persons with diabetes. They represent only a small sample of the hundreds and even thousands of dishes that are available in a plant-based macrobiotic diet. These dishes and remedies are not a complete meal plan but represent featured dishes in a broad-based and varied macrobiotic way of eating. Please consult the books in the Recommended Reading section for a more complete diet plan. Contact Berkshire Holistic Associates for more information.

BROWN RICE WITH MILLET

Good for slow steady release of glucose into the bloodstream. Millet is a specific for strengthening the pancreas, the organ that produces insulin.

1. Wash 2/3 cup of organic short grain brown rice by covering with water, rinsing, and draining the water. Repeat three times. Do the same for 1/3 cup of organic whole millet.
2. Place the washed grains in a pot with a tight-fitting lid.
3. Add a small pinch of sea salt and 1 ½ - 2 cups of spring water.
4. Cover and bring to a boil on a medium high flame.
5. When the grains come to an active boil, reduce the flame to low and cook for 50-60 minutes.
6. Turn off the flame and let sit for several minutes.
7. Remove from the pot with a wooden spoon and place in a serving bowl. Sprinkle each serving with Sesame Seaweed Condiment or prepared seaweed flake condiments (see below).

Brown rice, millet, and other whole grains can be cooked in a pressure cooker. After washing bring 1cup of washed grain to a boil in 1-½ cups of water and when pressure is up, place a flame deflector under the pot. Lower the flame and cook for 50 minutes. Brown rice and other whole grains can also be soaked prior to cooking.

DRIED DAIKON WITH CARROT AND ONION

Daikon aids in the discharge of fat and liquid, thus aiding in healthy weight loss and management. Carrot and onion are used in macrobiotic healing to strengthen and revitalize the pancreas. The naturally sweet flavor of this dish reduces the desire for refined sugar and artificial sweets.

1. Soak 1/2 cup of dried daikon for about 10 minutes or until it is soft. If the dried daikon has a very dark color and the water is also dark, discard the water. If the water is a light color, you may use it in the dish

2. Place the dried daikon (chopped if desired) in the pot and add enough water to cover.

3. Cut equal amounts of carrot and onion into thin slices. The amount of vegetables can equal the amount of daikon.

4. Cover the pot, bring to a boil, and lower the flame. Simmer for 20-30 minutes until the vegetables are tender.

5. Season lightly with shoyu (organic soy sauce) and cook until excess liquid evaporates.

AZUKI BEANS WITH SQUASH AND KOMBU

Azuki beans and kombu sea vegetable provide a slow steady release of glucose. They have been used for centuries to strengthen and vitalize the kidneys. Sweet fall or winter squash blends perfectly with the beans and sea vegetable. It strengthens the pancreas while easing the craving for sweets.

1. Wash and soak ½ cup of azuki beans with a 1-inch piece of kombu sea vegetable (optional) for several hours or overnight.

2. Place the kombu in the bottom of a pot and add chopped hard winter or autumn squash, especially kabocha squash.

3. Add azuki beans to the pot.

4. Bring slowly to a boil without covering the pot. Cover after 10 to 15 minutes.

5. Cook on a low flame until the beans become soft, about an hour or more. The water evaporates as the beans expand, so add water from time to time to keep the level constant.

6. Add a few pinches of sea salt or shoyu to taste.

7. Cover and cook for 15 to 30 minutes or until most of the water has evaporated.

8. Turn off the flame and let sit for several minutes before serving. Garnish with finely chopped scallion.

VEGETABLE STIR FRY

Vegetables such as onion, carrot, burdock, cabbage, and others used in stir-fries provide a good source of complex carbohydrate. They strengthen and vitalize the pancreas. This method of cooking helps activate energy. High quality olive or sesame oil is especially recommended. Sesame oil was used in traditional medicine to strengthen and protect the eyes.

1. Cut vegetables in thin slices. Leafy greens and thinly sliced onion, carrot, burdock can be sautéed separately or in various combinations.

2. Heat oil in a skillet. When hot, sauté the vegetables for several minutes. Gently stir with chopsticks or a wooden spoon. There is no need for vigorous stirring or constant mixing.

3. Season with a pinch of sea salt or organic shoyu.

4. Simmer for several more minutes, adding water if needed.

The vegetables should be crispy and colorful, cooked but not over cooked. Cooking times may vary depending on the vegetables being used. Root vegetables like carrot and burdock require a longer cooking time than green vegetables. Sliced tofu may be added for a classic stir-fry.

ARAME WITH ONION

Arame was traditionally used to strengthen the spleen, pancreas, and stomach. Adding vegetables to the dish enhances flavor and healing and energizing properties.

1. Wash and drain 1 cup of dried arame.

2. Brush a frying pan with a teaspoon of sesame oil and heat.

3. Add 1/3 cup of sliced onion and sauté for 2 to 3 minutes. (Carrot, dried daikon, rutabaga, sweet corn, or other vegetables may be added as well.)

4. Place the arame on top of the onion and add just enough water to cover the sliced onion.

5. Bring to a boil, turn the flame to low, and add shoyu to taste.

6. Cover and simmer for 20 to 25 minutes. Add more shoyu if needed.

7. Simmer for 5 to 10 minutes. Mix and stir until liquid has evaporated before serving. Garnish with finely chopped scallion.

SESAME SEAWEED CONDIMENT

Sesame seeds are good for eye health. Sea vegetables contain minerals that help alkalize the blood and strengthen the quality of insulin secreted by pancreatic beta cells.

1. Roast wakame sea vegetable in a dry skillet over a medium flame until dark and crisp.

2. Grind into a fine powder in a clay-grinding bowl known as a suribachi.

3. Roast an equal amount of washed and rinsed sesame seeds in the dry skillet over medium heat. Use a wooden spoon to gently stir the seeds to avoid burning. The seeds will begin to pop when ready and give off a nutty fragrance. Lower the flame toward the end of cooking.

4. Add the seeds while hot to the suribachi with the crushed wakame. Slowly and gently grind with the wooden pestle until each seed is thoroughly crushed.

5. Store in an airtight container and sprinkle on brown rice and other grain dishes.

PREPARED SEAWEED CONDIMENTS

Maine Coast Sea Vegetable Company offers a variety of prepared sea vegetable condiments, all of which add valuable minerals and iodine to the diet while having low sodium content. They include Dulse, Kelp, and Triple Blend Sea Vegetable Flakes. They can be used daily on whole grain and other dishes.

KANTEN

Kanten is a refreshing jelled dish that cools and relaxes the body and promotes regular elimination. Processed from red sea algae known as tengusa (also known as agar), it has natural laxative and fat-burning properties and can be used as an aid to weight loss. Is ideal for use in warm or hot weather. This basic kanten dish is made with apple juice. Persons on restricted diets due to advanced diabetes need to consult their health professional regarding the appropriateness of consuming fruit or fruit juice. Kanten made with powdered organic green tea, known as matcha, offers a therapeutic alternative to fruit or fruit juice kanten.

1. Place organic apple juice or cider in a saucepan and add kanten flakes. Stir to distribute evenly.
2. Bring to a boil and simmer until the flakes are thoroughly dissolved.
3. Continue to simmer on a low to medium flame for about ten minutes, gently stirring throughout.
4. Pour into individual cups or shallow bowls, ideally with two to three inches of hot kanten liquid.
5. Set aside or place in refrigerator until completely jelled (about 1/2-hour in refrigerator.) Serve as is. Eat as a snack between meals or at the end of a meal as dessert.

Fresh seasonal fruit, such as melon, berries; apple, pear, etc. may be added to kanten. Please select organic varieties.

—

Slice when needed and place fruit at bottom of cup or bowl. Pour hot kanten liquid over the fruit and jell as suggested above. Those on restricted diets due to advanced diabetes need to consult with their health professional regarding the advisability of consuming fruit or fruit juice.

UME SHO KUZU

Kuzu is a root starch thickener with strengthening properties. Umeboshi is a pickled plum with strong antibacterial, digestive strengthening, and alkalizing effects. Ume Sho Kuzu is a standard macrobiotic drink to strengthen digestion, restore energy, reduce inflammation, and help the body discharge acidity. It has a strong salty-sour taste.

1. Dissolve 1 heaping teaspoon of kuzu in 2 to 3 teaspoons of cold water.

2. Add 1 cup of cold water to the dissolved kuzu.

3. Bring to a boil over a medium flame, stirring constantly to prevent lumping, until the liquid becomes translucent. Reduce the flame to low.

4. Add the pulp of ½ to 1 umeboshi plum.

5. Add several drops to 1 teaspoon of shoyu and stir gently.

6. Simmer 2-3 minutes and drink hot.

Resources

Berkshire Holistic Associates, c/o Eastover Estate and Eco-Village, 450 East St., Lenox, MA 01240. Community-based nutritional counseling, lifestyle guidance, and practitioner referral service. A division of Planetary Health, Inc., a 501(c)(3) educational organization. Visit: www.BerkshireHolistic.com.

Planetary Health/Amberwaves, PO Box 487, Becket MA 01223, 413-623-0012, email: shenwa@bcn.net, www.planetaryhealth.com, www.amberwavesofgrain.org, www.makropedia.com. A grassroots network devoted to preserving amber waves of grain and keeping America and the planet beautiful. Sponsor of the annual Macrobiotic Summer Conference at the Eastover Resort in Lenox and the Online Macrobiotic Winter Conference. Visit: www.Macrobiotic SummerConference.com.

Macrobiotics Today/George Ohsawa Macrobiotic Foundation (GOMF), 1277 Marian Ave., Chico CA 95928, 800-232-2372, www.OhsawaMacrobiotics.com. A macrobiotic publisher and educational center on the West Coast.

The Barnard Medical Center combines medical care with the latest advances in prevention and nutrition to create a health care plan designed for each client. If you need to treat and reverse diabetes, heart disease, high blood pressure, or other chronic conditions, the Barnard Medical Center will help you revolutionize your health.

5100 Wisconsin Ave. N.W., Suite #401
Washington, D.C. 20016
202-527-7500
202-527-7400 (fax)

The Macrobiotic Online Course is the first of its kind course combining video, audio, print and live interaction; students around the world have the opportunity to study all facets of a plant-based macrobiotic lifestyle with Edward Esko, the Founder of the International Macrobiotic Institute (IMI.) The IMI Online Certificate Course is designed to enable students to gain ongoing benefit from their daily practice of macrobiotics while developing the knowledge and skill to guide and counsel others. www.internationalmacrobioticinstitute.com

The Culinary Medicine School is a center for healing, transformation, and awareness in Lee, MA. Founded and directed by Bettina Zumdick the CMS offers studies and workshops in culinary medicine, self-care, and private chef services. For information, visit culinarymedicineschool.com or contact Bettina at 413-429-5610.

Recommended Reading

Barnard, Neal D. *Dr. Neal Barnard's Program for Reversing Diabetes*. Rodale Books, Emmaus, PA, 2008.

Esko, Edward. *Macrobiotic Nutrition: A Guide to Sustainable Plant-based Eating,* IMI Press, Lenox, Mass., 2018.

Jack, Alex and Sachi Kato, *The One Peaceful World Cookbook*. BenBella Books, Dallas, Texas 00000, 2017.

Kushi, Aveline and Wendy Esko. *The Changing Seasons Macrobiotic Cookbook.* Avery Trade, 2003.

Kushi, Aveline and Alex Jack, *Aveline Kushi's Complete Guide to Macrobiotic Cooking.* Time-Warner, New York, New York, 1985.

Kushi, Michio and Marc Van Cauwenberghe, M.D. *Macrobiotic Home Remedies: Your Guide to Traditional Healing Techniques.* Square One Publishers, Garden City Park, New York, 2015.

Kushi, Michio and Alex Jack. *The Book of Macrobiotics: The Universal Way of Health and Happiness.* Square One Publishers, Garden City Park, New York. 2012.

Kushi, Michio. *The Do-In Way: Gentle Exercises to Liberate the Body, Mind, and Spirit.* Square One Publishers, Garden City Park, New York. 2009.

Kushi, Michio. *Your Body Never Lies: The Complete Book of Oriental Diagnosis.* Square One Publishers, Garden City Park, New York. 2010.

Zumdick, Bettina. *Authentic Foods.* 2012.

NOTES

---

[1] Michio Kushi and Alex Jack, *The Book of Macrobiotics*, Tokyo and New York: Japan Publications, 1985.

[2] F. M. Sacks, Bernard Rosner, and Edward H. Kass, "Blood Pressure in Vegetarians," American Journal of Epidemiology 100:390-98, 1974. F. M. Sacks et al., "Plasma Lipids and Lipoproteins in Vegetarians and Controls," New England Journal of Medicine 292:1148-51, 1975. F. M. Sacks et al., "Effects of Ingestion of Meat on Plasma Cholesterol of Vegetarians," Journal of the American Medical Association 246:640-44, 1981. William P. Castelli, "Summary of Lessons from the Framingham Heart Study," Framingham, Mass., September, 1983.

[3] U.S.D.A., *Dietary Guidelines for Americans*, 2000.

[4] B. R. Goldin et al., "Effect of Diet on Excretion of Estrogens in Pre- and Postmenopausal Incidence of Breast Cancer in Vegetarian Women," *Cancer Research* 41:3771-73, 1981. James P. Carter et al., "Hypothesis: Dietary Management May Improve Survival from Nutritionally Linked Cancers Based on Analysis of Representative Cases," *Journal of the American College of Nutrition* 12:209-226, 1993. Miriam S. Wetzel et al., "Courses Involving Complementary and Alternative Medicine at U.S. Medical Schools," *Journal of the American Medical Association* 280:784-87, 1998. "Complementary and Alternative Therapies, American Cancer Society Internet Site, 1997; "Alternative and Complementary Therapies," *Cancer* 77(6), 1996. Franco Berrino et al., "Reducing Bioavailable Sex Hormones through a Comprehensive Change in Diet: the Diet and Androgens (DIANA) Randomized Trial," Cancer Epidemiology, Biomarkers, & Prevention 10: 25-33, January 2001. Macrobiotic Research Project," Jane Teas, Ph.D., principal investigator; Joan Cunningham, Ph.D., co-principal investigator, sponsored by the Centers for Disease Control, October 2000 to September 2002, University of South Carolina, Prevention Research Center, School of Public Health, Charleston, S.C. www.macrobiotics.sph.sc.edu/project.htm. "Guide for Nutrition and Physical Activity for Cancer Survivors," *CA: A Cancer Journal for Clinicians*, Sept-Oct. 2003. R. Kaaks, "Effects of Dietary Intervention on IGF-Binding Proteins, and Related Alterations in Sex Steroid Metabolism: The Diet and Androgens (DIANA) Randomized Trial," *European Journal of Clinical*

Nutrition 57(9):1079-88, 2003. G.A. Saxe et al., "Potential Attenuation of Disease Progression in Recurrent Prostate Cancer with Plant-Based Diet and Stress Reduction," *Integr Cancer Ther* 5(3)206-13, 2006.

[5] J. Bhjumisawasdi et al., "The Self-Reliant System for Alternative Care of Diabetes Mellitus Patients—Experience Macrobiotic Management in Trad Province," *Journal of the Medical Association of Thailand* 89(12):2104-15, 2006.

[6] Carmen Porrata, M.D., PhD., et al., "Ma-Pi 2 Macrobiotic Diet Intervention in Adults with Type 2 Diabetes Mellitus," *MEDICC Review*, Fall 2009, 11(4):29-35.

[7] Robert H. Lerman, M.D., Ph.D., "The Macrobiotic Diet in Chronic Disease," *Nutri Clin Prac* December 2010; 25(6):621-626.

[8] N. D. Bernard et al., "A Low Fat, Vegan Diet Improves Glycemic Control and Cardiovascular Risk Factors in a Randomized Clinical Trial in Individuals with Type 2 Diabetes," *Diabetes Care* 2006; 29:1777-83.

[9] N. M. McKeown et al., "Whole-Grain Intake Is Favorably Associated with Metabolic Risk Factors for Type 2 Diabetes and Cardiovascular Disease in the Framingham Offspring Study," *American Journal of Clinical Nutrition* 76(2):390-8, 2002.

[10] L. N. Panlasignui and L. U. Thompson, "Blood Glucose Lowering Effects of Brown Rice in Normal and Diabetic Subjects," *International Journal of Food Science and Nutrition* 57(3): 151-8, 2006.

[11] B. J. Venn and J. I. Mann, "Cereal Grains, Legumes, and Diabetes," *European Journal of Clinical Nutrition* 58(11):1443-61, 2004.

[12] Min Sun Kim et al., "Effects of Seaweed Supplementation on Blood Glucose Concentration, Lipid Profile, and Antioxidant Enzyme Activities in Patients with Type 2 Diabetes Mellitus," *Nutrition Research and Practice* (2008), 2(2):62-67.

[13] Maeda H., Yamamoto R., Hirao K., Tochikubo O.. "Effects of agar (kanten) diet on obese patients with impaired glucose tolerance and type 2 diabetes." *Diabetes Obes Metab.* 2005 Jan;7(1):40-6.

[14] F. Fallucca et al., "Gut microbiota and Ma-Pi 2 macrobiotic diet in the treatment of type 2 diabetes," *World Journal of Diabetes* 2015 Apr15:6(3): 403-411.

[15] M. Candela et al., "Modulation of gut microbiota dysbioses in type 2 diabetic patients by macrobiotic Ma-Pi 2 diet," *British Journal of Nutrition*, 2016 May 6:1-14.